Meloxicam

A comprehensive guidebook that teaches readers about nonsteroidal anti-inflammatory drugs used to treat the symptoms of osteoarthritis and arthritis

Dr. Tyler K. Kevin

Table of Contents

Chapter One

Introduction to Meloxicam

Millions of people throughout the world suffer from arthritis and osteoarthritis, two prevalent musculoskeletal illnesses that cause persistent pain and diminished joint function. Meloxicam stands out as a key participant in the effort to control the symptoms of these incapacitating illnesses among the variety of therapeutic options available.

Nonsteroidal anti-inflammatory medications (NSAIDs), which include meloxicam, are known for their effectiveness in reducing pain and inflammation. Meloxicam stands out due to its specific suppression of inflammatory enzymes. By concentrating on these particular offenders, Meloxicam provides a twofold benefit that can considerably improve the quality of life for people with arthritis and osteoarthritis by reducing pain while also addressing the underlying cause of joint inflammation.

In order to treat these illnesses, Meloxicam main goal is to bring about much-needed symptomatic relief. Whether you struggle with the lingering pain of osteoarthritis or the inflammatory flare-ups typical of rheumatoid arthritis, Meloxicam can be a trusted ally. It reduces discomfort, making it possible to resume everyday activities more comfortably. Additionally, by reducing inflammation, Meloxicam helps to maintain joint functionality and may reduce the advancement of these disorders, reducing the chance of additional damage.

Development and Approval History of the Drug

The tale of Meloxicam development and approval is a monument to medical researchers' perseverance and dedication to making the lives of people with chronic pain and inflammation better. Meloxicam, which is frequently regarded as a pharmaceutical milestone, has a long history that dates back to the late 20th century.

Pharmaceutical companies set out to develop a new class of nonsteroidal anti-inflammatory medications (NSAIDs) in the late 1980s that would be able to relieve pain with fewer gastrointestinal side effects, a common worry regarding existing NSAIDs. This project resulted in the development of Meloxicam, a drug with strong anti-inflammatory effects and a good safety profile.

Meloxicam efficiency in lowering pain and inflammation, especially in illnesses like arthritis and osteoarthritis, was established in clinical trials carried out in the early 1990s. During the drug's development, it underwent extensive research to determine its safety, effectiveness, and any potential side effects. Meloxicam has the potential to meet the unmet medical needs of those with chronic musculoskeletal pain, according to researchers and healthcare professionals.

In 1994, regulatory agencies in numerous nations started approving the use of Meloxicam as a prescription drug following considerable research and clinical testing. With the potential to replace current NSAIDs, its release onto the pharmaceutical market was an important turning point in the field of pain management. Meloxicam gained popularity as time went on because it had a reputation for being more effective at relieving pain than certain other NSAIDs while also having less gastrointestinal problems.

Chapter Two

An Explanation of Osteoarthritis and Arthritis

Millions of individuals throughout the world suffer with arthritis, a general term for a number of inflammatory joint illnesses. It's critical to understand that arthritis is a series of connected conditions rather than a single illness marked by joint pain, stiffness, and inflammation. The name "arthritis" itself is derived from Greek terms that mean "joint" and "inflammation," indicating the defining characteristic of these illnesses.

Osteoarthritis is frequently referred to as "wear-and-tear arthritis" because it normally progresses slowly over time as a result of the progressive destruction of joint cartilage. The cartilage that cushions the ends of bones in a joint deteriorates over time, which causes pain, stiffness, and decreased joint function. Although osteoarthritis can affect any joint in the body, it most frequently affects the knees, hips, hands, and spine. Given that it tends to get worse with age, this ailment is more common in older people.

Another prevalent type of arthritis is rheumatoid arthritis, which differs greatly from osteoarthritis. Rheumatoid arthritis is an autoimmune condition, in contrast to osteoarthritis, which primarily impacts joint cartilage. In this illness, the synovium, a membrane lining the joint capsules, is mistakenly attacked by the immune system. In addition to harming the synovium, this ongoing inflammation also causes the bone and cartilage in the joint to break down. Rheumatoid arthritis can strike at any age and frequently affects several joints, resulting in edema, discomfort, and abnormalities of the joints.

The choice of treatment modalities, including the potential use of drugs like Meloxicam, depends on an understanding of the differences between these two common types of arthritis. Rheumatoid arthritis requires therapies that inhibit the immune system to reduce inflammation and prevent joint destruction, while osteoarthritis often calls for measures to ease symptoms and limit progression.

Prevalence, Reasons, and Risk Factors

A significant fraction of the world's population suffers from arthritis, which includes several different types of joint inflammation. Its widespread occurrence is evidence of the substantial influence it has on people's lives and healthcare systems around the world. Even though specific numbers may vary by geography and demographics, arthritis poses a serious public health threat.

One of the most common types of arthritis, osteoarthritis, primarily affects older people, although it can also affect younger folks. Osteoarthritis is one of the top 10 most incapacitating diseases in developed nations, according to the World Health Organization (WHO). Osteoarthritis is thought to affect millions of people each year and is the most common cause of pain and disability. The prevalence of osteoarthritis is predicted to increase as the world's population ages, highlighting the need for powerful medications like Meloxicam.

Osteoarthritis has a number of multifactorial reasons, many of which are yet unknown. But a number of things influence its growth. Age-related joint deterioration and mechanical stress are important factors. Furthermore, genetics can affect a person's propensity to develop osteoarthritis. People who have certain genetic variants may be more susceptible to joint issues. Obesity, joint malalignment, and joint traumas are additional risk factors. People who work in or engage in activities that put a lot of strain on particular joints are also more vulnerable.

Rheumatoid arthritis, on the other hand, is an autoimmune condition, which means that the immune system unintentionally targets the body's own tissues. Millions of people around the world are affected by it, and it affects people of all ages, including kids. Although the precise etiology of rheumatoid arthritis is unknown, it is thought to be a result of a mix of genetic, environmental, and hormonal factors. Rheumatoid arthritis risk has been associated with smoking and several infections.

It is essential for both patients and healthcare providers to comprehend the prevalence, causes, and risk factors connected with arthritis and osteoarthritis. It assists in the development of effective treatment alternatives like Meloxicam, early diagnosis, and preventative initiatives.

Chapter Three

An Explanation of How Meloxicam Reduces Pain and Inflammation in the Body

A non-steroidal anti-inflammatory medicine (NSAID) called meloxicam works wonders by specifically targeting the body's pain- and inflammation-producing enzymes. It's critical to explore the complex mechanics underlying these activities in order to comprehend how Meloxicam functions.

A natural response of the body to injury or infection, inflammation is frequently characterized by redness, swelling, heat, and discomfort. But in diseases like arthritis and osteoarthritis, this defense mechanism malfunctions, causing chronic inflammation and unbearable agony. Cyclooxygenases, or COX enzymes, are the key players in this inflammatory response.

The main mechanism of action of meloxicam is to sparingly affect COX-1 while significantly reducing COX-2 activity. Prostaglandins are lipid compounds that play a critical role in modulating pain and inflammation. COX-1 and COX-2 are the enzymes in charge of creating these lipid compounds. Assisting in blood clotting and stomach lining defense are only two of the regular bodily processes that COX-1 is involved in sustaining. However, COX-2 is primarily linked to the inflammatory response.

By specifically inhibiting COX-2, Meloxicam lowers the levels of prostaglandins—which are involved in causing pain and inflammation—that are produced. Meloxicam is able to relieve the pain brought on by arthritic and osteoarthritis conditions while retaining vital COX-1-mediated functions thanks to this focused strategy. Meloxicam is a powerful and well-liked option for controlling pain and inflammation in these diseases because of the delicate balance it strikes between reducing pain and maintaining physiological processes.

People can select the administration strategy that best meets their needs thanks to the fact that meloxicam is offered in a variety of formats, including pills, capsules, and oral suspension. Meloxicam major objective is to lessen pain and inflammation, which can have a serious negative influence on the lives of people with arthritis and osteoarthritis. This objective is the same whether the drug is taken orally or applied topically.

Comparison with Other Non-Steroidal Anti-Inflammatory Medicine

Meloxicam belongs to the same class of drugs as many other nonsteroidal anti-inflammatory drugs (NSAIDs) that are sold in the market. Meloxicam special qualities and unique position in the field of pain relief and inflammation control, however, are what distinguish it from other medications.

The COX-2 enzyme, which is principally in charge of causing inflammation and pain, is selectively inhibited by Meloxicam, which is one of the drug's key differentiators. The COX-1 enzyme is more significantly spared thanks to Meloxicam selective action, which enables it to focus on the underlying causes of discomfort. As a result of this COX-1 sparing, many other conventional NSAIDs carry a lower risk of gastrointestinal side effects, which is a common worry. Meloxicam may prove to be a more secure and comfortable long-term pain management alternative for people who are more prone to stomach irritation or bleeding.

The COX-2 selectivity and risk of adverse effects of various NSAIDs varies in comparison. Older NSAIDs like ibuprofen and naproxen are less selective, affecting both COX-1 and COX-2 enzymes, which increases the risk of gastrointestinal problems. These drugs work well to reduce pain and inflammation, but they might also need to be used for a short period of time or with gastro protective medicines to lessen the risk of unwanted side effects.

Meloxicam also has a longer half-life than many NSAIDs, making it possible to take just one dose per day, which makes it easier to follow treatment plans and more convenient. This is particularly advantageous for people who need long-term pain management for illnesses like osteoarthritis or rheumatoid arthritis, when constant, daily dosing is necessary for the best symptom control.

While Meloxicam has special benefits, it's crucial to remember that selecting an NSAID should always be based on a patient's particular needs, medical history, and a healthcare provider's suggestion. Certain illnesses or patient profiles may respond better to certain NSAIDs than others.

Chapter Four

Guidelines for Recommended Dosage and Administration

Understanding and following the suggested dosage and administration parameters are crucial for the efficient and secure use of Meloxicam. Important information is provided in this area to help people get the most out of this drug while reducing any dangers.

Meloxicam standard beginning dose for adults is 7.5 milligrams (mg) administered once day. Under the guidance of a healthcare practitioner, the dosage may be raised to 15 mg per day in some circumstances, particularly when a higher analgesic effect is required. Excessive dosage can increase the danger of adverse effects without adding any additional benefits, thus it's critical to adhere to the appropriate dosage exactly as given by a healthcare professional.

Meloxicam can be taken with or without food, however taking it with food, especially a meal or a snack, may help lessen the chance of stomach trouble. A full glass of water should be consumed along with the medication, which is normally taken orally in the form of tablets or capsules. The tablets should not be broken, chewed, or crushed because doing so could change how the medication is supposed to be released.

To maintain a constant level of the medication in the bloodstream, Meloxicam should be taken consistently at the same time each day by people with rheumatoid arthritis or osteoarthritis. Its effectiveness may be impacted if you deviate from the recommended schedule.

If a dose is missed, patients shouldn't take two doses at once; instead, they should take the next dose at the usual time. A double dose can result in an overdose, which could have negative repercussions.

To effectively treat symptoms, Meloxicam must be taken for the least amount of time possible. Long-term use should be closely monitored by a physician, and medical professionals may periodically reevaluate the necessity for ongoing therapy.

People should never self-adjust their Meloxicam dosage or discontinue taking the medicine abruptly without first talking to a healthcare provider. This could have negative effects and increase the risk of pain and inflammation returning.

People can take full advantage of Meloxicam ability to manage the signs and symptoms of arthritis and osteoarthritis while upholding their safety and wellbeing by following these dosage and administration recommendations. It is crucial to get individualized advice from a healthcare professional as different medical situations and histories can affect the right dosing schedule.

Conditions and Signs for Which Meloxicam is Recommended

A versatile drug called meloxicam is typically used to treat diseases marked by pain and inflammation, especially those that affect the joints. It is an effective therapy choice for a variety of medical disorders due to its ability to reduce these symptoms.

One of the most prevalent diseases for which Meloxicam is recommended is osteoarthritis, sometimes known as "wear-and-tear arthritis." Due to the slow destruction of joint cartilage, it typically affects older persons. People can restore mobility and enhance their quality of life thanks to meloxicam ability to relieve the pain, stiffness, and inflammation that come along with this condition.

Rheumatoid Arthritis: An autoimmune condition known as rheumatoid arthritis causes chronic joint inflammation and destruction when the immune system assaults the synovium inadvertently. Meloxicam is an effective component of the rheumatoid arthritis treatment plan, assisting in the reduction of pain and inflammation and possibly delaying the course of the illness.

Joint pain and swelling are symptoms of juvenile idiopathic arthritis, which affects children and teenagers. Juvenile patients who are suffering from the symptoms of juvenile idiopathic arthritis may occasionally be given meloxicam, which improves joint function and relieves their pain.

Ankylosing Spondylitis: The spine is the main area of the body affected by this form of inflammatory arthritis, which results in stiffness and discomfort. Meloxicam can be a beneficial part of therapy regimens for people with this condition, helping to control their symptoms and improving spinal flexibility.

Painful Menstrual cycles: Meloxicam may occasionally be administered to lessen the suffering brought on by dysmenorrheal, or painful menstrual cycles. Its anti-inflammatory characteristics can aid in reducing discomfort and cramping throughout the menstrual cycle.

Meloxicam may also be used to treat several other inflammatory disorders, such as tendinitis or bursitis, in which pain and swelling are the main symptoms. It could be a component of an overall therapy plan to ease discomfort and speed up the healing process.

It's vital to remember that Meloxicam is only recommended under the supervision of a medical practitioner, who will evaluate the particular disease, its severity, and the patient's unique health profile to determine whether the prescription should be used. To get the best benefits while lowering any dangers or side effects, it's essential to follow the dose instructions and dosing schedule exactly.

Chapter Five

Meloxicam Use's Potential Negative Effects and Risks

A person should be aware of any possible hazards and side effects before using meloxicam, just like with any medicine. Despite the fact that Meloxicam is generally well tolerated by most users, it is important to be aware of and educated about these possible side effects.

Effects on the Digestive System: Meloxicam and other nonsteroidal anti-inflammatory medicines (NSAIDs) can have adverse effects that affect the digestive system, which are among the most often reported side effects. These side effects can include gastrointestinal bleeding or ulcer development in more extreme circumstances, along with stomach pain, indigestion, and nausea. The risk of these problems can be decreased by taking Meloxicam with food or as directed by a healthcare professional. A preventive medicine regimen may also be necessary for people with a history of stomach ulcers or gastrointestinal bleeding.

Cardiovascular Risks: Some studies have speculated that NSAIDs, including Meloxicam, may be associated with a marginally elevated risk of cardiovascular events including heart attacks and strokes. People who already have heart issues or who are at risk for developing them may be at higher risk. These variables are taken into account by medical professionals when recommending Meloxicam, and those who are at higher risk may also be given the choice of alternate treatments.

Renal function: Meloxicam may have an impact on renal function, particularly in people having kidney disease already. During prolonged use, it might be required to regularly check renal function. To maintain kidney health while using Meloxicam, it's imperative to drink plenty of water.

Allergic Reactions: Although uncommon, Meloxicam allergic reactions can happen. Hives, itchiness, swelling (particularly of the face, lips, tongue, or neck), extreme wooziness, or trouble breathing are all indications of an allergic reaction. Seek emergency medical assistance if any of these symptoms appear.

Liver Function: In very rare circumstances, meloxicam may have an impact on liver function. Dark urine, persistent nausea, and abdominal pain are all signs of liver issues. Jaundice (yellowing of the skin or eyes) is another. Any odd symptoms should be reported to a healthcare professional right once.

Additional Potential Side Effects: Meloxicam may also cause headache, sleepiness, dizziness, and fluid retention. High blood pressure, heart failure, or blood abnormalities could be less frequent but more severe adverse effects. If these adverse effects manifest, medical assistance is necessary.

It's critical to take Meloxicam under the supervision of a medical expert who can examine your unique health profile and balance the dangers and benefits. Your medical history, current medications, and any underlying illnesses will all be taken into account as they decide on the best course of treatment for you. People who use Meloxicam should follow the dosage and instructions exactly, report any strange symptoms right once, and go to frequent checkups to have their health monitored.

Chapter Six

Precautions and Contraindications for Meloxicam

To ensure its safe and efficient usage, people and healthcare professionals should be informed of the risks and contraindications that come with meloxicam, a nonsteroidal anti-inflammatory medication (NSAID).

Allergies: People who are hypersensitive to or allergic to meloxicam or other NSAIDs should refrain from using it. Hives, swelling, itching, and difficulty breathing are just a few of the signs of allergic responses, which can be quite serious.

Meloxicam may raise your chance of developing gastrointestinal issues like ulcers, bleeding, or perforation. Meloxicam should be used with caution by those who have a history of stomach ulcers or gastrointestinal bleeding, and they should talk to their doctor about additional safety measures, like gastro protective drugs, before starting the prescription.

Cardiovascular Health: Meloxicam has been linked to a modest increase in the risk of cardiovascular events, such as heart attacks and strokes, particularly in people with prior heart diseases or risk factors. Before administering Meloxicam, medical professionals must carefully evaluate each patient's cardiovascular risk profile; for patients with higher cardiovascular risk, alternative medications might be recommended.

Meloxicam can impact the function of the kidneys and liver. Long-term users, especially those with kidney or liver illness already present, may need to have regular checks on their organs' health. Maintaining kidney health requires drinking enough water.

Asthma: Taking Meloxicam may raise the risk of asthma exacerbations in people with a history of the condition. Such people require constant observation and the right kind of management.

Meloxicam should not be used during pregnancy or while nursing since it may cause issues for both the mother and the unborn child, especially during the third trimester. Avoid using it right before giving birth. A breastfeeding infant may be harmed by Meloxicam if it enters breast milk. When evaluating its use while pregnant or nursing, healthcare professionals will carefully compare the risks and advantages.

Individuals over the age of 65 and those in poor health may be especially vulnerable to Meloxicam side effects, including gastrointestinal bleeding and cardiovascular problems. For this demographic, lower doses or alternate therapies may be thought about.

Drug Interactions: Meloxicam may have an effect on the way that other drugs work or increase the likelihood that adverse effects will occur. All medications, including over-the-counter medicines and supplements, should be disclosed to a healthcare professional by a patient.

In conclusion, meloxicam is an effective drug for treating pain and inflammation, but it should be used with caution, especially in people with certain medical disorders or risk factors. Before beginning Meloxicam, it is crucial to address any current health issues with a healthcare professional. They can give you individualized advice on how to use it safely and effectively. To monitor health and reduce potential hazards, it is essential to follow the dosage instructions and checkup schedule provided by a doctor.

Chapter Seven

Answering Common Questions Regarding Meloxicam

1. Is meloxicam a prescription drug or is it available over-the-counter?

A: A prescription is normally required to purchase meloxicam. It's critical to seek medical advice from a professional who can assess your health history and decide whether Meloxicam is the best course of action for your particular problem. They will also recommend the appropriate dosage and offer instructions on how to use it safely.

2. Is it safe to combine meloxicam with other NSAIDs or painkillers?

A: Generally speaking, taking Meloxicam with other NSAIDs or painkillers increases the chance of adverse effects, especially gastrointestinal problems. The risk of harmful cardiovascular events can also increase when NSAIDs are combined. To prevent potential interactions, it's crucial to let your healthcare practitioner know about all of your prescription and over-the-counter medications, as well as any supplements you use.

3. How long does it take Meloxicam to begin to work?

A: The time it takes for Meloxicam to start working varies from person to person and is influenced by a number of variables, such as the level of pain or inflammation, the ailment being treated, and how well the patient reacts to the drug. While some people may find relief within a few hours, others could need several days of regular use before noticing any real changes.

4. I take Meloxicam; may I drink alcohol?

A: In general, it's best to minimize or forego alcohol when taking meloxicam. The risk of gastrointestinal adverse effects, such as stomach bleeding or ulcers, which are already connected to the use of NSAIDs, can be increased by alcohol. Alcohol and Meloxicam usage together may increase the risk of liver and renal issues.

5. Is using Meloxicam for an extended period of time safe?

A healthcare professional should supervise the long-term usage of meloxicam. While controlling chronic disorders like arthritis can be safe and successful, it's crucial to keep an eye out for any potential adverse effects and to often determine if further treatment is necessary. Based on your unique medical condition and how the drug is working for you, your healthcare professional will decide on the right amount of time to use it.

6. If I forget to take a Meloxicam dose, what should I do?

A: If you forget to take a dose of Meloxicam, do so as soon as you remember, unless it is almost time for your next dose. You should then skip the missed dose and resume your regular dosing plan.

To make up for a missed dose, do not take two; doing so increases the possibility of experiencing negative side effects.

7. Can I use Meloxicam if I've had stomach ulcers or gastrointestinal bleeding in the past?

A history of stomach ulcers or gastrointestinal bleeding must be disclosed to your healthcare professional. Meloxicam can be used, however there may be additional safety measures that are needed, such as the co-prescription of gastro protective drugs to lessen the risk of stomach discomfort. The ideal strategy for your circumstances will be determined by your healthcare practitioner.

8. Can kids and teenagers used Meloxicam ?

A: Children under the age of two should not typically take meloxicam. Its administration to children and teenagers should be done with the help of a healthcare professional because the safety and dosage may change depending on the child's age, weight, and particular medical condition.

9. Do people using Meloxicam have to follow any dietary restrictions?

A: Meloxicam use does not come with any specific dietary restrictions. The risk of stomach discomfort might be minimized by taking it with food or a snack. It is typically advised to support overall health when using Meloxicam by eating a balanced diet and drinking plenty of water.

10. If I have a history of high blood pressure or heart problems, is Meloxicam safe to take?

A: People who have had heart disease or high blood pressure in the past should use Meloxicam with caution. A modest rise in the risk of cardiovascular events has been linked to NSAIDs, especially Meloxicam. Your healthcare professional must be informed about your medical history in order to properly assess the risks and benefits of the proposed course of treatment and, if necessary, seek alternative course of treatment alternatives.

Made in the USA
Las Vegas, NV
02 January 2024

83789421R00024